Blessed *in the* Midst *of* Trial

Sarah,
As you go through this journey, may your eyes always be open to the blessings around you. God's blessings upon you!
W

ERIK JELINEK

Blessed *in the* Midst *of* Trial

Cancer, Chemo, & Keeping the Faith

TATE PUBLISHING
AND ENTERPRISES, LLC

Blessed in the Midst of Trial

Published by Tate Publishing & Enterprises, LLC
127 E. Trade Center Terrace | Mustang, Oklahoma 73064 USA
1.888.361.9473 | www.tatepublishing.com

Tate Publishing is committed to excellence in the publishing industry. The company reflects the philosophy established by the founders, based on Psalm 68:11,
"The Lord gave the word and great was the company of those who published it."

Cover design by Kate Stearman
Interior design by Sarah Kirchen

Published in the United States of America

ISBN: 978-1-61346-590-5
1. Biography & Autobiography / Personal Memoirs
2. Religion / Christian Life / Inspirational
11.09.27

This is dedicated to my wonderful wife, Jennifer,
and our girls, Sierra and Scarlett.
You provided me the love, hope, and support
needed to make it through this journey

And to the doctors who have been
God's hands in my life:
Dr. Miller, Dr. Patel, Dr. Weigel,
Dr. Vogel, and Dr. Mahler.
It is because of you and your staff that
I was able to write this book.

The "C" Word? Really?

My wife and I were sitting in the doctor's office, waiting for our appointment. He was running a little late, so we just sat there, thinking too much and saying very little.

Finally he came in. I introduced him to Jennifer, and then he sat down and looked at me.

"The good news," he said, "is that we know what it is. The bad news is it is what we feared."

Cancer.

Age thirty-eight, a nonsmoker, and I had lung cancer. At that moment it felt like the world was collapsing around me. I thought of Jennifer, my wife. I thought of our two girls, ages five and one. I thought of everything I wanted to do and hadn't yet. I thought of milestones that I might miss. I thought the worst about what could happen.

Cancer. One word, but in saying it everything changed.

Amazingly, though, it was the blessings that came through this disease that caused me to see that face of

God more clearly than I ever have before because of all the people I saw God working in and through.

Throughout my life I have been quite blessed. I grew up in a great family with my mom, dad, and sister being wonderfully supportive. I actively participated in a variety of sports, especially football and track. I had great friends with whom I have maintained friendships, and I was blessed to have a strong education and a love for learning that has not abated over the years.

I am married to Jennifer, my best friend and the light of my life. We live in southern Wisconsin, where we are both pastors at a Lutheran church. We have two little girls who keep us running and invite us to see the blessings of life in new ways as we get the opportunity to see the world through their eyes. Yes, I have seen blessing upon blessing throughout my life.

But it has been through this trial, this valley in the road of life, that I have begun to see blessings in a new way. You see, the blessings that I have had in the good times in life do not even compare to the blessings that I have been showered with through the struggles in life. This story, my story, is about my greatest trial to date in life and how, every step of the way, there have been blessings poured out upon me—blessings in ways, and through people, that I never would have expected.

A Headache Becomes a Blessing

On the first day of March, I had a regular checkup with my doctor. I had been feeling great. I was getting more exercise, I was sleeping a little better, and spring was on its way. So life was good—I just had to get a checkup, and I was off for another six months. I had these regular checkups because I have cluster headaches, and we were trying different things to minimize the pain that comes with them. Cluster headaches are like migraines, only worse. I normally have one "cluster" a year, and it lasts for about six weeks. During this time I can get up to two headaches a day. These headaches can incapacitate me and can take anywhere from ten minutes to three hours to dissipate. So the purpose of these checkups was to see how the headaches were going and if there was anything new to try. What a blessing that I had these headaches, for it opened the door for healing to take place.

My primary care doctor came in, and we talked about how things were going. She gave me a little checkup, and then she asked about the walking pneumonia I had six months earlier.

"I feel great. There is no wheezing anymore. It looks like the meds cleared it all up," I said.

"That's great," she responded. "But to be on the safe side, let's do a chest CT. Just to see how the lungs are recovering."

Okay. A little test then I can get out of here. "Let's do it."

So I went downstairs, did the paperwork, had some dye shot into my body, and was scanned. For someone who was not a fan of medical tests, this one was not too bad.

That night my doctor called.

It is never a good thing to have your doctor call you at home.

"Erik, it looks like you probably have some scar tissue on your lungs. I have arranged for you to meet with a pulmonologist on Wednesday, and most likely he will run a few tests to make sure."

What could I say—another doctor and maybe another test. *Let's do it and be done.*

Wednesday I met with the new doctor. He reviewed everything and said, "Yes, it looks like scar tissue, but to make sure it is not an infection I want to do a PET scan."

Oh joy, I thought, *another test, and this time I have to lie in a tube. I hope they have some good meds for this, because that is going to be tight.*

As you might have guessed, I am not a fan of confined spaces.

And they did have good meds. Two days later, at the hospital again, and this time I was given a drug to relax.

Jennifer had dropped me off and would be back later to pick me up. So I had to lie in a room for an hour to let the dye go to work. Then they wheeled me to a machine where I put my hands above my head, and they scanned my entire body. Not a lot of fun, but the drugs did their job, and I left feeling okay about the whole thing.

I then walked out to meet with Jennifer, and off we went for the night. I would not have results for a few days, so we went about our regular work and family business over the weekend.

Monday I met with the doctor again, and this time he told me that it wasn't scar tissue because the PET scan showed that it was active. He still thought it was an infection, but he wanted to make sure. So he recommended a bronchoscopy, and he would biopsy what was in there.

Great. Another test. And this time they are going to shove a tube down my throat.

So two days later I was back at the hospital. Again. Jennifer dropped me off at seven a.m., and I went through all the paperwork, changed into one of those wonderful hospital gowns, and was given a few shots and an IV.

Two hours later I was wheeled into the procedure room. They gave me a med that would wipe out my memory of the event. After that my eyes were covered with a cloth.

I remember the tube entering my mouth and a slight cough. The next thing I knew, the doctor was asking me who the president was.

Another test done. I was so hoping this would be the last.

Friday morning, two days later, I was with Jennifer in the doctor's office. That was when we got the news that floored both of us.

I was too young. I was too healthy. Yes, I could stand to lose a few pounds, but still.

Cancer.

Tears That Bring a Clearer Sight

During this time I never went to the "why-me" questions. It might have had something to do with the fact that a few weeks earlier Jennifer had preached on that subject, or it might have had something to do with the shock I was in. But I never asked why me. I wept. I cried out to God. I struggled. But it only took a few days for me to see the first of many blessings.

My doctors found the cancer.

That is the first big blessing here. I had a primary care doctor who saw something that looked a little strange, and she decided to pursue it. From what I now understand, many doctors would not have done anything with these tests for at least a year, but not my doctor. No. She was moved to do more tests, and because she did, the cancer was found. Because the cancer was found, I was able to start the healing process—wherever that led me. As you may imagine, I truly love this doctor. For her to make the time, to do the follow-up, to even call me at home and check in with me after I received the news—she is a phenomenal doctor and an even better person.

So, yes, a blessing happened in the form of diagnoses, and God's hand was clearly at work through this doctor who decided to take the next step, follow her gut, and find out what it was that looked odd to her on that test.

It reminds me that even in the most trying of situations, we are not walking alone. We have the blessings of loved ones, the blessings of professionals who know what they are doing, and the blessings of a God who loves us and walks every step with us. Even when we stumble, when something comes our way that is not what we expected or what we wanted, we still have God there to support us. When our eyes are opened to the love he has for us, we then are able to see his face shining through, surrounding us, and reminding us that we are loved, cared for, and needed. Yes, we are all precious in God's sight, and as his beloved children, our eyes are opened to the blessings he showers on us. These are blessings that abound even in the darkest of times, the times we hear the words we fear and wander into dark valleys that appear to have no end.

After first hearing the devastating news, we knew we had to tell a number of people—our family, our friends, and, as pastors, we had to somehow tell the congregation. So Jennifer and I went to work. She went home to tell family, and I went to the office to tell the staff, family, and a few parishioners.

That was hard.

I never expected to have to walk into the office and say, "I have lung cancer," but it had to be done. I told the staff one by one. I called family and friends. I got in touch with a friend who is an assistant to the bishop and let him know as well. A few minutes later, the bishop called me. It was when I was on the phone with the bishop that I first really lost it. I had shed some tears in the doctor's office when I was told, but it was on the phone with the bishop, trying to explain what had happened, that I got very choked up and even tried to get off the phone as fast as I could because I knew I was losing it. I was losing it because for the first time it felt real. It felt like this could be the end, and I was not ready for that to happen. This was the first of many times over the next few months that I would lose it.

But it was also during this time, when I was weeping, that I heard my own advice to others come back to me: It is okay to cry. It is okay to be emotional. It is okay to weep and cry out to God. God's shoulders are big enough to handle your pain, so let him. And I did.

I then sent e-mails to others. Piece by piece I did what needed to be done. Looking back on it, I was just operating without any real sensation. I knew what had to happen; I knew who had to be called. The word had to get out, so I got it out.

And then came the night.

After all the calls. After going home and having dinner with my family. After kissing the girls and tucking them in for the night. Then came the night. And I lost it. Again.

I remember lying there in bed, watching Jennifer come out of the bathroom, and I just lost it, wondering if I would have a chance to see my girls grow up. Yes, the emotions had to come out, and this time they came out like a torrential storm. I never asked why but instead what will happen? What will happen to the girls? What will happen to my wife? What will happen to me? Am I going to live to see another year, or is this it? Will I watch my girls graduate? Will I be there to walk them down the aisle? Will I grow old with my wife? Will I have the chance to retire with her, or will I not even make it that far?

The questions poured through my mind, the tears flowed down my cheeks, and the emotions bubbled out of me. It was a long night.

That weekend I was supposed to preach, but Jennifer took over. We both knew it would be too hard for me to make the announcement and preach, so I stepped out of the pulpit. At the Saturday evening service, I came forward at the beginning and announced that after a series of medical tests it had been discovered I was unique—a young, nonsmoker with lung cancer. Everyone was shocked.

I had to do the same announcement three more times on Sunday morning. Each time very few people knew what to say to me except "I am sorry," and "I will be praying for you." At the end of the last service, one of the members came up and said, "Now you are gaining more information for sermons. Think of everything you can tell us after you beat this." That stuck with me.

That night we traveled to see Jennifer's family. Everyone was still in shock. But it was a very strange sensation to be sitting in a room with family and friends, thinking how I had a tumor growing inside me and had to be cut open in order to live. This is not something most people think about.

But it was also here when something started to click. Something happened that night. The Spirit was blowing, and my ears just happened to be open. For, once again, I started to see the blessings. To see how lucky I was.

God's Breath Gives New Vision

The Spirit moves in strange and wonderful ways, and that night as the Spirit blew across me, my eyes were opened to the blessings of what had just happened.

As I mentioned, my doctor—the one I went to see for a semiannual checkup—decided to run a test that many doctors would not have considered. I didn't have any symptoms of illness at all. Yet she decided to run the test. She decided to do a little bit more digging all because something just didn't feel right with her. If she hadn't done that, the cancer would have grown, and the situation might have been much worse than it was. In reflection, she was the first blessing.

The second blessing that came to me that night was the pulmonologist. Here was a doctor who was pretty sure he knew what I had, but he needed to be positive. So he ran a test, and even when that came back, he thought he knew what it was, but still he wouldn't stop. He had to know, so he ran another. What a blessing he did because it was that last test that confirmed the cancer. It was that last test that said it was a good thing we did all this because we could operate. If he hadn't, well, who knows? The cancer might have grown so big that it was inoperable, and the treatments might have been more for pain management instead of treatment. But that was not the case, and I was blessed to know I had cancer and had it at a treatable stage.

Yes, the Spirit is a strange and wonderful gift. For in the blowing of the Spirit across our lives, we are brought into contact with people who fill us with blessings. It may not be the doctors who find something that is well hidden, and it may not be something that is life or death. It may be the Spirit opening you to see the needed word of a neighbor, the caring hand of a loved one, or a shoulder to lean on.

As we continued down this road, the blessings continued.

By this time I had been informed that I was operable and I had a meeting set up with a surgeon in Madison. So while I was waiting to meet with her, they started me on some pre-op tests with the assumption that the surgery would be fairly soon.

So the next week there were two tests to endure—a stress test and a breathing test. I was oh so excited.

First up: the stress test. I headed off to the clinic and was led into a room where they shaved a few patches on my chest, put on some sensors, and said, "When the doctor comes in, you step on this treadmill and run. Many people think they can run on here as long as on a regular treadmill, but you can't. This was designed to work you very hard and make you stop soon."

Now I was excited.

In came the doctor, and off I went. Three minutes, and the grade and speed of the treadmill changed.

Six minutes. Now it was steeper and moving faster.

Nine minutes. Okay, this was not fun anymore.

Twelve minutes. I was really hoofing it. The sweat was pouring down me. The treadmill was steeper than I normally climb on a hike in the mountains. Everything was moving so fast.

Thirteen minutes. I was done.

Thirteen minutes, I thought, *at least I was in double digits.*

So they sat me down, went through everything, and said, "The record here is held by a seventeen-year-old soccer star. He went seventeen minutes. You did great."

Relief flooded over me—my heart was good enough for surgery. It is not that I ever doubted it, but the affirmation was a blessing in itself.

Next stop was the breathing test, and that happened a few days later. I met up with the same nurse who did the brochoscopy. It turned out that she had been on vacation since the last time I saw her, so I got to inform her about what had happened with me since then. She then told me about the type of surgery she thought I would have. Then she made me empty my lungs.

These tests actually are not as bad as they sound. I got a little lightheaded after one or two of them, but overall it was pretty easy. I was then informed that I did not have to do the last few tests because my lung capacity was at 123 percent.

Again, I was ready for surgery. But here is also where some frustration set in. I was healthy. My stress test showed a very healthy body. The breathing test showed very healthy lungs. Yet there was something inside me that could kill me. It was in my lungs. In that part of my body that seemed to be doing so well.

If I only felt sick. If I only had trouble breathing, or a wheeze, or anything that would show that I had this tumor in me. But I didn't. Which, in hindsight, I see again as a blessing because if I did have symptoms, it would mean that the cancer had progressed much further and recovery would be more difficult. But then it was frustrating being told I was sick and not feeling it.

When I was younger, I was extremely active. I was in at least three sports a year. I ran, lifted weights, did everything a person could possibly do to stay in shape. Over the years some of my activity dropped off due to work schedule, family life, and, more often than not, just the excuses I came up with. I always told myself I would get back to the exercise, and sometimes I would for a few months, but then I would slack again.

Nonetheless, my body has decent muscle memory, and because of the exercise I did in my younger years, even though I was overweight, my body was still quite healthy. Because of this blessing and the early discovery even though the cancer did not want to show itself, I was going to beat the cancer.

Yes, the blessing is that I was healthy—healthy enough to have surgery, healthy enough to recover quickly, healthy enough to have the strength to go after every cancer cell that might be hiding in me and wipe all of them out.

That was the plan.

And after all of these pre-op tests, it was time to put the plan into action.

God's Healing, Human Hands

But before surgery could take place, I had to meet two more doctors: the oncologist who would be treating me after the surgery and the surgeon who would open me up and take these poisoned cells out of me.

My first meeting was with the oncologist.

I truly admire oncologists. These are doctors who have devoted their lives to fighting a disease that claims way too many lives. They are on the front lines and have to deal with people who are truly struggling and in pain. The one I met was a man who is filled with constant faith as he does his amazing work.

He came in and we went over my latest scans. He showed me where the tumor was and discussed how he thought this was caused by a genetic mutation. He also reassured me, saying he knew my surgeon and thought she was top notch. After the surgery I would be seeing him again to set up chemo and radiation schedules. He also talked about getting an MRI to see if the cancer had spread, but I tried to bypass that part of the conversation because I really did not want to think about the MRI or spreading cancer. Then, before he left, he did something that surprised me.

He asked to pray with us.

Earlier in the conversation, he had asked about what I did for a living. When I told him that both my wife and I were pastors in town, he took the information down and kept going with the conversation. But now he felt comfortable enough with us that he offered to pray with us.

Another blessing—a doctor who was willing to be open about his faith and pray with two people he'd just met, knowing we were scared and unsure of what the future might hold for us.

So we prayed.

After the prayer there was a sense of peace, a sense of comfort that this would work out, that I was in the right place with the right doctors and nurses, doing what needed to be done in order to beat this cancer and live that life I have been blessed with to the fullest.

The next day I was scheduled to meet my surgeon and part of her team. I had done a little bit of research on her and found out she was one of the top cardio-thoracic surgeons in the United States. She specialized in lung cancer surgeries and wanted to wipe out as much cancer as she possibly could.

I also realized that being one of the top cancer surgeons in the United States meant that she was very, very busy. We were scheduled to meet with her and the team on Wednesday at 3:30 in the afternoon. I had invited a friend,

Nancy, to come with us because she is a retired doctor and could help interpret anything we might not understand.

We also decided to take two cars to the meeting, which turned out to be a blessing. All of this was happening during Lent, and we had Wednesday evening services that night. So to be on the safe side, Jennifer would have a car and could leave if the meeting was running late.

And the meeting was late. Very late. Our appointment that was scheduled for 3:30 p.m. started around 7:00 p.m. Nearly four hours in a waiting room filled with cancer patients and their families is not fun.

Since the meeting was running so late, Jennifer could not stay. She had to get back and lead worship. This was tough for a number of reasons: First, waiting that long to meet with the surgeon was frightening. There was the fear of the unknown, the fear that the cancer had progressed too far, the fear that she would say that there was nothing she could do. Second, Jennifer was not able to meet the one who was going to open me up and start the healing process for me.

But Nancy stayed, and this was a blessing as well, for she was able to keep me calm and relaxed as we waited.

Then there was yet another blessing: when we finally met with this surgical team, the first person we met was one of the surgeon's fellows. This was another top-notch doctor who had amazing talent and was easy to get along with. He brought into the room a sense of hope.

This doctor went through all of the scans again. He talked about what the surgery would look like, how long it would take, and what the recovery process would be like.

Any question we had he answered. He was in no hurry to get anywhere—I also think we were the last meeting of the day—and he wanted us to be comfortable with everything. Finally he asked, "So when do you want to have the surgery?"

My response: "Now!"

He left and came back in a few minutes with the surgeon. When she entered I could tell she knew what she was doing. She opened up the scans again and pointed out the tumor and other issues that needed her attention. She then talked about the surgery—how there were two possible ways of doing it. The first would be to cut three little holes in my side and remove the right upper lobe of my lung through those holes.

The second option would be used if they could not get everything they wanted the first way. They would cut a six-inch incision under my armpit, spread my ribs, and take out the lobe of my lung and as many lymph nodes as possible through that incision.

The preferred method would be the option with the three holes, but the team would not know which they would perform until they got into surgery. Another incredible blessing would come out of this.

Then, after all this explanation about what would happen to me, the surgeon did something that no one, no doctor, up to this point had done.

She said, "This is treatable."

Until then the word *treatable* had never been uttered. We were hopeful. We thought we had caught it early enough. But none of the doctors had said anything about being treatable.

This doctor, this surgeon who specialized in lung cancer surgery, had just said the cancer was treatable.

That I was treatable.

It didn't stop there. She then said that I was in the top 20 percent of the people she sees. She said it looked like a stage-three cancer, but I was in the top 20 percent because it was restricted to one area in my lung. I learned that cancer is often categorized into four different stages, with stage one being the most confined and easiest to treat while stage four is the most progressed and hardest to treat.

Then she said, "I do have some bad news though. The earliest we can do the surgery is April 15." That was three weeks away.

My thought was, *If this is the bad news, that I have to wait three weeks to surgery, I am truly blessed here.*

They assured me that in the life of cancer, three weeks is nothing. The tumor was not going to grow that much, and in three weeks they would be doing the same thing that they would have had done if the surgery was today.

She informed me there would be a few more tests that would need to take place, including an MRI. The purpose of the MRI was to make sure the cancer had not spread into the brain. With my fear of tight spaces, I tried to talk my way out of this test but to no avail. So the following week I was scheduled to travel to Rockford, Illinois, where they had an open MRI machine, and then go back to Madison to meet with one of the team members and do my pre-op.

Another week and two more tests, and then I would be done until the surgery. That was a good thing because Sierra, our oldest daughter, was getting tired of having Daddy go see the doctor so much. This was another one of the struggles that we faced, trying to let a five-year-old know that Daddy was sick and would have to go to see a lot of doctors and eventually spend a few days in the hospital. Sierra is a very bright girl, and she knew something was going on, so one night I sat down with her on the couch and said, "You know that Daddy has been seeing a lot of doctors lately, right?"

"Yes, Daddy, and I want you to be done," she replied.

"Well, honey," I said, "there is something inside Daddy that shouldn't be there. It could make Daddy very sick. So Daddy is going to see a few more doctors, and then he is going to have to spend a few days in the hospital because they are going to take the bad thing out of him. And when Daddy comes home, then you cannot jump on him for awhile."

"Oh," she said, "but when you get better I can jump on you again, right?"

"Right," I said, laughing, "when Daddy is better, you can jump on him."

She understood enough at the time. We also told her teacher and daycare leaders in case there were some problems down the road. But throughout this whole thing, she has been wonderful and helped in many ways—with me, with Jennifer, and with her little sister, Scarlett. She even helped make a chemo care kit.

I cannot say enough good things about all of the doctors that I have encountered on this journey. All these people have been blessed with healing hands and compassionate hearts and are more than motivated to make others better. It is through them that I have seen the hand of God at work, and they are so motivated to help and heal others.

Then there is the blessing of family. Without family it would have been extremely easy to slip into a hole of despair and stay there. But having Jennifer as a pillar of support kept me going through some of the more difficult times. Her love, her compassion, her encouragement is what was needed to remind me that through all of this there is life. And life is so much more than just existing as you go through a struggle. Life is reaching out with both hands and embracing every moment that comes your way, knowing that in that moment, good or bad, Christ is walking with you and showering you with the love and compassion that is needed. This love, this self-giving, unending love is embodied in my wife, and because of her I could see the joy of living every day.

And then there is the blessing of the girls. Sierra and Scarlett bring such joy to a room that it is nearly impossible to be in a bad mood when they are running around and playing. They reminded me that life keeps going. Even when we have to slow down and rest for awhile, life keeps going. Their full-speed, run-at-all-costs energy blessed me with the insight to see how life is to be enjoyed and treasured every step of the way.

I Really Have to Go Into That Tube?

There were two sets of tests left before the surgery—the MRI and the pre-op work. First on the list was the MRI.

I really did not want to do this test, and I had two good reasons in my head.

Reason number one: I really dislike enclosed spaces. I don't like caves, tunnels, tubes, anything that encases me. I am not sure where this fear comes from, and I really have no desire to find out, but the MRI was one of my great fears. I did find an open MRI in Rockford, so that was where I would do the test.

Reason number two was more personal. What if they found a tumor in my brain? What if the cancer had spread? If either of these were answered with a yes then the surgery would be off, and my life expectancy would have just plummeted. In my wonderfully warped brain, the thought was *If I do not do the test, then they cannot prove the cancer has spread.*

But my two specialists both insisted on the test. So down I drove to Rockford, thinking about the test. I had been told that it would take close to two hours to do the whole thing, and I was wondering how crazy I would drive myself, just lying there and thinking for two hours.

Ah, and here came the blessings again. It is truly amazing to see how many blessings have been poured out on me throughout all of this.

After signing in and getting all of the insurance information down on paper, I met the technician, and she was wonderful. She had me change into a skimpy little gown and then brought me into the room with the MRI machine, which was quite cold. She had me lie down, and immediately I felt better about the test. On this table I was able to have my arms out to my sides, and even though I had a facemask on and was inches away from the MRI plate, I was comfortable. So I was able to close my eyes, talk with God, and think some very positive thoughts.

As we were getting near the end of the tests, I had about twenty minutes left, according to the technician, who spoke to me over the PA system in the room. She said, "I wanted you to know I am not a radiologist, but from what I see everything looks great. There are no tumors here."

Here was another one of those blessings. According to the technician, the one who does this three or four times a day, there was no tumor. The cancer had not spread. I was still treatable. I was still operable. I was truly blessed.

The rest of the test went quickly. I then drove home, calling everyone I could and letting them know that the MRI had been a success.

The following Monday I met with part of the surgical team again, and this was the final meeting before surgery. I also knew that if anything weird had shown up on the MRI, I would be hearing about it here as well.

The pre-op went extremely smooth. All of the test results were above average. Everything looked great. I was walked through the procedure one more time and then told that I would get a call the day before the surgery to know what time to be there. My goal was to have the first surgery of the day, to get the surgeon just as she was starting out.

Then I was done. In four weeks I had a dozen different doctor's appointments and tests, and now I was done until the surgery.

It was a little strange, not having to run from appointment to appointment. But it also gave me the opportunity to settle back into my "normal" life. And it just happened to be the start of Holy Week. There could not be a better time for me to focus on faith and what God went through for us. I entered that Holy Week with a very different focus than I had any year before, or any year for that matter.

I am a big-picture person. I enjoying looking at where I am, where the church is, and seeing where we could be in the next five, ten, or fifteen years. I can see past little details to big panoramic pictures and find ways to make those pictures come to life.

Having said that, I do not do well with the normal and mundane. I always want to be on the move. I always want to be envisioning the future and finding ways to make it a reality. I would not be a good chaplain, doing the same thing day after day. It would wear on me way too much.

But I did come to realize a major blessing during this time as well: the blessing of a normal and mundane week.

After all the tests and running back and forth from different hospitals and clinics, being able to slow down and have a normal week opened my eyes to the blessings of the regular day. During this time I could get Sierra ready for school, have a cup of coffee, and enjoy my devotional time, not feel rushed to make it to an appointment, have lunch with my wife, and simply enjoy the people I interacted with during the day.

It was the blessing of the normal, the blessing of the basic gifts in life—something I may have realized but did not truly treasure until now.

Life, Death, and Life Again

In the life of the church, Holy Week is the busiest week of the year. This is the time when we reflect upon the final week of Jesus's life, what he endured, and the blessings he showered upon us through his trials, death, and resurrection.

It is also the week when we have the most services. We celebrate Palm Sunday with the triumphant march that Jesus makes into Jerusalem, waving palms and singing our Hosannas. It is a joyful celebration that takes a dramatic turn halfway through the service when we read the entire passion narrative and hear of the last days of Jesus's life.

The next service at our church is on Maundy Thursday. This is the day we sit with Jesus and the disciples in the upper room and share in his last meal. It is a night of learning about service and how we are called to care for others by watching Jesus wash the feet of his disciples. We also celebrate the institution of the Lord's Supper—the body and blood of Christ being poured out for us as we hear those powerful words, "Given and shed for you for the forgiveness of sin."

It was also the first time that I was back in the pulpit since learning about the surgery. This was not an easy sermon for me to give. But as I was preparing for the service, my eyes were opened once again, and I was able to see the body of Christ, that is, the church, in action. One of our staff members had started working with her mother on setting up a care team for me and my family. They already had people lined up to help with yard work, meals, and babysitting. These were things that we had not thought about, but the church did them.

So the sermon focused on love—the love we have been blessed with by God and the love that we share with one another.

Not long after I became a father, a friend gave me some advice. He said, "Your children will be your greatest joy and your greatest challenge. They will make you smile and cry on the same day. They will fill your heart with joy, and your heart will break when they stumble and fall. But there is one key to being the best dad that you can be—love them. Just love them."

These words have echoed in my head over and over throughout the years: love them, just love them. For it is in that love, in that wide embrace of grace, that relationships are built, restored, and flourish. It is in that love, that life-giving love, that the face of Christ shines through and we are given a glimpse of the glory of God.

Maundy Thursday is all about love. It is about the love that Christ demonstrates for his disciples and us. It is about the love that flourishes in this body known as the church. It is about the love that we are called to share.

Love them, just love them.

And it all starts with an ordinary little action. You see, Jesus uses this ordinary action, the washing of feet, to demonstrate an extraordinary love. And he calls his disciples, he invites you and me, to do the same.

Back in Jesus's time, people commonly washed their own feet. When guests arrived at someone's home with feet covered in dust from the road, a good host would offer them a basin of water. The host would not do the washing but would provide the water so that the guests could wash their own feet. In some cases the host would have a slave wash the feet of the guests. But it was understood that no free person would stoop down to wash the feet of another free person. Hospitality meant offering water and perhaps the services of a slave. It did not mean doing the washing.

For a free person to wash someone else's feet meant that he or she was taking on the role of a slave. The only reason someone would do this was to show complete and utter devotion to another person. That is what Jesus does here.

He assumes the role of a slave to show the depth of his love for his disciples. Love them, just love them, and he does this by serving them. And his love does not stop here.

No, Jesus continues to live out the love he has for us by inviting us to share in a meal. He gathers with us at a table.

He breaks some bread. He lifts a cup, and he says to us, "This is me.

"This is my body, this is my blood. This is what gives me life. And when you eat and drink of this, when you share in this meal, it will give you life, too."

Yes, in this meal we are given the strength that we need to make it through all trials or struggles we may be facing. We are given the gift of knowing that the God who called us by name, the God who claimed us as his own, is also the one who showers us with grace and forgiveness. Yes, God is the one who wipes away our sins, cleanses us, and empowers us to go out into this world that he has created and live as little Christs for others.

Love them, just love them.

Yes, Jesus does this. He loves us by giving his very being to us and reminds us every time we share in this meal he is present. He is here. Through his body and blood, he is recreating, forgiving sins, and creating a new life in each and every one of us. Talk about love!

He then loves us, just loves us, by encouraging and calling us to community building. You see, in telling the disciples to wash one another's feet, in calling us to share in a meal, and in commanding us to love, to love as he has first loved us, as we hear at the end of the gospel reading, Jesus is inviting us to be about community building (John 13:1–17, 31b-35).

For in the serving of each other, in the eating with each other, in the loving of one another, a community is created. A community that we now call the body of Christ. And it is in this body that the love of God is reflected. Reflected to those gathered here and reflected to those who are not yet a part of the body. Reflected to all of creation.

As I dealt with the surprising news of my cancer diagnosis, the talk of treatments, and what all this might mean for me and my family, I have been blessed to see this love, this amazing love, with new eyes. With all of the struggles, with all of the sorrow, with all of the questioning and the crying out, God has spoken to me through this great body of his. This has forever enhanced the way I see this Maundy Thursday. For I have seen the love and service of Christ shared with me and my family by the congregation I am blessed to serve as pastor. In prayers, cards, and the wonderful hugs. I have gathered at this table with this great body. Shared in the meal that promises to bring hope and healing. Knowing that I gather with others who are struggling as well that we all gather to receive that body and blood that we so desperately need. And I have experienced the love, the life-giving love of Christ, for I have seen his face, and I have seen it in this congregation I am honored to call "family."

Love them, just love them.

That is the mantra of Maundy Thursday. A mantra of love, a mantra of compassion, a mantra of new life.

What If?

Holy Week was a tough time for me in 2010. I felt blessed that the surgery was not until after Holy Week. In fact we were going to be able to take a family vacation before the surgery. But that meant more time to think about the surgery.

It also meant more time to reflect on what Holy Week meant to me. It was a very personal journey that I was taking that year because everything seemed to have more significance.

Sitting at the table with the disciples, watching the trial on Good Friday, walking to Golgotha with Jesus as he carried the cross, hearing the nails as they were pounded in and Jesus was lifted up high, seeing him take his last breath.

It was powerful that year. More powerful than in previous years. I think it was this way because I had been given an up-close and personal view of my own mortality. This cancer could kill me. We were not sure exactly how far it had spread, and there was the possibility, as there is with any cancer, that it had spread farther than was treatable. Everything was in our favor at this time, but still, it was cancer, and that made me nervous.

So on that Holy Week, as I went through all the steps with Christ again, I could not help but think, *What if this is it? What if this is the last Holy Week that I get to celebrate? What if next year I am resting in the arms of Christ?*

It was a difficult three days. But then came Sunday, Easter Sunday.

As I rose that morning to prepare for the sunrise service, it hit me. The power of that Easter Sunday hit me head on, and I was overwhelmed with blessings again.

For it is exactly because we do not ever know when it will be our last Holy Week, our last Easter, our last day here on earth, that Easter has such a great significance in our lives. For it is because of what Christ did, it is because of his death and resurrection, that we are able to rest in the fact that new life is born. Yes, new life is born on this Easter morn, and it is born in each and every one of us, for God died so that we may have life and have it eternally.

Yes, that Easter morning was different than any of the other Easter mornings I have celebrated. It was more powerful because of the realization of my mortality. It was more powerful because of the time I spent pondering the blessings I, and all of God's children, have been given by Christ. It was more powerful because I was looking at Easter with new eyes, with eyes filled with gratitude for all that God has blessed me with.

Easter turned out to be a true blessing that year. The services were filled with wonderful music, and the Spirit could be felt in a very tangible way. I also was enjoying Easter more than I had in the past because I was of the mindset that I did not want to take any moment for granted. I wanted to celebrate each and every moment I had, and so, on that Easter morn, I celebrated the promises that Christ made for me, for you, and for all of his children.

Then, as the morning came to an end, it was time for a break. A break from work, a break from medical tests. A break to prepare myself mentally and physically for the next stage of this process. So, on Easter Sunday afternoon, we went on vacation.

Every year after Easter we go on vacation. It is our annual recover-from-Lent-and-Holy-Week vacation where we recharge our batteries, get to spend time with family, and normally go somewhere warm to shake off the Wisconsin chill of winter.

This year we were going to meet Jennifer's family in Florida. They make an annual pilgrimage to a place on the panhandle, and we had gone with them a few times in the past. This year was different though because we had decided to drive. It was going to be an interesting trip, to say the least.

It went well. We drove through the night so that the girls could sleep in the back of the van. We tried to sleep when not driving, but that did not go quite as well. Jennifer has trouble sleeping in vehicles, and my mind was racing—*Is this the last family vacation I will go on? How can*

I make it memorable? What is there for me to do in order to make this the best vacation ever?

I actually put a lot of pressure on myself, but as the drive progressed, once again I was hit by the Spirit.

It doesn't have to be the perfect vacation. It doesn't have to be the most memorable event ever. All it has to be is what it is: a vacation with family, a time to relax, and an opportunity to spend time with people I love without the pressure of work, meetings, and doctors' appointments.

That is what it turned out to be—a wonderful break. We swam, played on the beach, rested, relaxed in the sun, and went for long walks that were needed for health of body and soul. Jennifer and I even had a date night one evening. We saw a really bad movie, but it was a nice night out anyway.

On the way home we took our time and drove through Nashville and Indianapolis. We stopped at the children's museum in Indianapolis and had a wonderful time with the girls. By the end of the trip we were ready to be home, but we all had a great time.

Plus, I was rested for the next stage of the journey. When I had met with my surgeon, she recommended we take this trip because she thought the next four months would be very difficult. I felt good about all the family time and the rest I had gotten on the trip, so I was ready. Ready to have the surgery, ready to have the cancer removed from me, ready for the next stage of the journey.

The Healing Begins

We got home on Sunday night, so I had until Thursday to get everything in order before the surgery. The girls got back into their regular routine, and Jennifer and I prepared the best we could at church for the time we would take off.

It was also at this time that I saw the blessings of the church come shining through again. The care team, which I knew so little about, was in full swing. They had gotten Jennifer some gift cards to use for meals when she was visiting me in the hospital, as well as gas cards for driving to and from Madison. There was a list of people set to take care of the girls, and meals were going to be coming to the house as soon as I was checked out of the hospital.

On Tuesday night we had a special service at church as well. We had a healing service where we encouraged everyone in the congregation who was struggling to come for a time of prayer and laying on of hands for healing. We asked a pastor in a neighboring congregation to come and lead the service, and our congregation board president assisted her as well.

We had told the other pastors in the area what we were doing, and the majority of them showed up too as a sign of their support and to add their prayers to all of the others that evening.

It turned out to be one of the most emotional services I have been a part of in my ministry. Mary preached a moving sermon on the healing touch of God, and when it came time for the laying on of hands, she invited people to come forward to the altar rail. She also invited other people in the congregation to come and lay hands on those who were asking for prayers as well.

We went forward, Jennifer and I, and kneeled down at the altar rail. I heard some rustling behind me but did not look up. When it was our turn and Mary laid her hands on me, she invited the others behind me to lay their hands on me as well.

I thought there were only one or two people behind me. There weren't.

No, instead there were over a dozen people lined up behind me. All of them laid their hands upon me and Jennifer or on the person in front of them. And as Mary prayed I could just feel the Spirit coursing through all of the people gathered there.

God was at work. He was at work through his body, through his church. He was going to shower his blessings upon everyone he could because that is what God does—blesses his children.

It was a moving night and a wonderful foretaste of the rest of the week.

On Wednesday I got in touch with the hospital in Madison and found out that I was indeed the first surgery of the day. The surgery would take place at 7:20 a.m., which meant that I needed to be there by 5:30 a.m. to get prepped for the surgery. Instead of trying to leave at four in the morning, we decided that we would get a hotel room that night to make the morning a little bit easier.

That night I taught a confirmation class. It was the first one we had in a few months because of the Lenten services, so the youth came with their parents to talk about what they had learned in the past month. But the majority of the time was spent talking about me, the surgery I was about to have, and what the cancer meant to me, my family, and the church.

Again, I saw the blessings of the church in this meeting, for the students and parents expressed an interest in helping any way that they could. They also knew they could ask me anything about what was happening, and I would answer as honestly as I could.

After confirmation I met up with Jennifer at home. Her mother had come down to take care of the girls, so we gave them kisses goodnight and then drove up to Madison. We checked in by 10:00 p.m. On the drive up there I thought it was going to be a long, sleepless night with me thinking about the surgery and tossing and turning all night long, but luckily that was not the case. Instead we were both out in a matter of minutes. This was another one of those blessings where our bodies knew the stress we had been under and the rest that we needed, so we crashed and crashed hard.

The next morning we were up early, checking out before most people were even close to being awake. We made it over to the hospital and checked in at the surgery desk just before five thirty a.m. We then went and sat with the half dozen other people who were waiting to have surgery.

At this point I knew that two people were going to try to come and see me before surgery. The first was a friend, Pedro, who worked in the bishop's office. He had e-mailed earlier in the week to find the time for the surgery and said he was coming to pray with us before I went in. I also had a friend, Mitch, who had traveled in from Minnesota to sit with Jennifer during the surgery. We knew he had made it into town, and we thought he would show up before the surgery as well.

At 5:30 a.m. the nurse came and got all of us who were scheduled for surgery to line up. We then were escorted to little curtained-off rooms where they gave me one of those wonderful backless robes and told me to change into it. After I had changed and put everything I had into a bag I gave to Jennifer, the nurse came back and started taking all my vitals, put in an IV, and went over everything with me.

I had been told earlier that the surgery would be anywhere between three and five hours long. The plan was to knock me out and then do another brochoscopy to see if they would open me up with only three small incisions and take out the lobe and lymph nodes thorascopically or if they would have to do the six-inch incision to remove everything. It all had to do with where the cancer was located and what they might find once they got in there.

After that they would turn me on my side and make the incisions that were needed, take out what they could, then close me up. That was the plan.

After the nurse reviewed everything with me, she asked if I had a power of attorney and living will signed. I did and gave it to her to put on file. *Always better to be prepared,* I thought.

Then the anesthesiologist came in, and he explained everything they were going to give me and how it would be administered. He got another IV going, asked if I had any questions, and went to get ready.

Then Pedro came. This was a wonderful blessing, for in the midst of the craziness of getting prepped for surgery, Pedro came and brought a little piece of peace with him. We talked about the surgery, he shared some scripture, and he prayed with us.

Once again I was reminded of the blessings of being a part of the church. For here I was, a pastor, being ministered to by another in a time that was very stressful and frightening. To have others to gather with, pray with, and support, was a blessing in itself.

Then we got word that Mitch, our friend from Minnesota, had arrived. So Pedro excused himself, and Mitch came in. He was there only a minute, and in came the surgeon.

This was the first time that Jennifer had met the surgeon, since the first meeting had been so late and she was unable to stay. So the surgeon introduced herself, went through a few things, then said, "It's almost time. So say your good-byes, and we will be on our way soon."

At that point, the rest of the surgical team came in. I said good-bye to Jennifer and gave her a little kiss. Then she left, and I was wheeled out of the little room. I was taken down a long white hall and told that I only had a few things that I needed to do from this point on. I was going to have to help move my body off of the bed onto a steel operating table, and I was going to have to lie back after I got on it. *Easy enough,* I thought.

So I was wheeled into the operating room, and the bed was lined up with steel table. I helped hoist my body from one bed to the other. Then I felt my feet being strapped down. And that was it.

That is all that I remember from the surgery.

Next thing I knew, I was propped up on a bed, and they were pulling me forward to slip a metal plate behind my back. I looked up and saw that they were taking an X-ray of my lungs. I scanned the room and saw a number of other people reclined in beds, all in various stages of grogginess. This was the recovery room. I told the nurses that I was thirsty, and they gave me some ice chips to suck on. It is amazing how good ice chips can taste. It is a sensation I will never forget. The cold, the wet—it reminded me I was alive.

A few minutes later, I was told they were coming to move me up to my room. So they took all the stuff I was hooked up to and loaded it on the bed. Then we went wheeling out of the room and into a hallway. Again, the memories here are a little shaky, but soon I was being wheeled into a room. I looked up, and there was Jennifer.

What a wonderful face to see.

She came into the room with me as they were adjusting everything and making sure all the monitors were working. Over her shoulder in the hall I saw three friends, including Mitch. They waited out there until I was settled.

I also looked up at the clock in my room and it read 2:35 p.m. Now this confused me. The surgery was supposed to be three to five hours long and then an hour in the recovery room. That would make it between eleven and one, not 2:35. So I said to Jennifer, "It took a little longer than expected."

She said, "Yes, it did."

Then I asked, "What happened?"

"I think I should wait to tell you until you are less heavily medicated," she replied.

"No, tell me now." I said.

"Okay," she said, "When they were about to close you up, they found another tumor in your chest. It was a different type of cancer, and it was on your heart. They had to run some tests on it before they could remove it because they wanted to confirm that it was a different type of cancer. The doctor also said that even though it was the size of a ping-pong ball, she was not worried about it. She will tell us more when she comes up later."

What a way to wake up from surgery by being told that not only was part of my lung removed, but there was a second tumor that had been on my heart. But again, almost immediately, I saw the blessing here as well.

You see, it turns out that when they did the bronchoscopy at the start of the surgery, they determined they should do the larger incision rather than make the three little cuts and use the scope. They then went in and took out the right upper lobe as planned. They scraped the lower lobe to make sure that the cancer had not spread. They removed eleven lymph nodes to have them tested, knowing that some would come up positive.

It was then, after they were done and were about to close, that they saw the tumor on my heart.

They would not have seen this if they had not made the large incision. It would have been missed and still sitting in there.

What a blessing that they opened me up as they did. What a blessing that I had doctors who took the time to look around and see the tumor and then remove it.

It was hard on Jennifer during that time. She had to sit and wait a number of extra hours, not knowing what was going on, especially at the end. But again there are blessings here. For not only was Mitch there, but two friends had popped by to check on her as well. The blessing of community shone through on that day.

As I adjusted to the news of the second tumor, the doctors and nurses continued to get me settled. At this point I started to feel a major pain in my back. It felt like a huge muscle cramp that just would not go away. They put a hot pack on my back with the hopes that it would take care of it. This muscle cramp stuck with me for over two weeks after the surgery, and it turned out it was there because of the way they positioned my body during the surgery.

The reason I bring up this pain is that it was the only real severe pain I had after the surgery. Yes, there were a number of uncomfortable moments, there were a few times when I moved wrong and my side hurt, but overall this muscle cramp in my back was the worst pain I had.

Again, another blessing—the pain was not as bad as I expected it to be.

After I was settled in the room, my friends came in to say hi. One of them left their coffee on the edge of the bed, a big mistake as the nurse bumped it and spilled it all over the bed. So it didn't take too long to get new sheets.

After an hour or so, some of the drugs had worn off, so I was allowed to have my phone and check e-mail as well as Facebook. I did my first post-surgery Facebook update about two hours after surgery. It said, "Wow—it feels like they cut my side and pulled out something—oh wait they did—ahh morphine button."

Ever since I was diagnosed, I had been doing postings about the cancer and doctors' appointments on Facebook and on my blog. One of the main reasons I was doing this was to keep the congregation and family and friends who lived out-of-state informed as to what was going on. The response I had received during this time was overwhelming. People from all over the world were praying for me and sending greetings and uplifting stories of people they knew who were survivors. It lifted my spirits. So when I posted after the surgery, I was once again overwhelmed with the support and love that I felt from friends all over the world.

Within two hours the nurses had me up and walking. The most difficult part of that process was getting out of bed. I was hooked up to an IV and had a chest tube, so I had to push the IV and carry the box attached to the chest tube. But once I was up and going, I felt great. At that point I decided that every time I got up, if it was to change from the bed to the chair or go to the bathroom, I would go for a walk as well. This paid off in spades because my recovery time in the hospital went very quickly.

That night I had a light dinner as we waited for the doctor to come and talk to us. The nurse told us that the doctor normally had a full day of surgery on Thursdays, and today she was running behind schedule, so she would not be in anytime soon. Finally Jennifer left to go home to the girls, and Mitch headed out to the hotel so I could get some sleep. About midnight the doctor finally came in. She had just finished her last surgery of the day (remember mine was at 7:20 a.m.) and she was checking in on her patients. Her first question to me was "Why are you still awake?"

She then filled me in on the surgery. It turns out that she was very aggressive during the surgery, and it was a good thing she was. That was why she found the other tumor on my heart. She also told me she thought I was stage three B because of the size of the tumor and the number of lymph nodes they took, but that would be checked out later, and at a post-op meeting I would learn more. Then she was off to see another patient.

I am continually amazed at the blessings I received during this entire time. This surgeon decided to make the larger incision and because of that found an extra tumor that needed to come out. Because of her experience, the gifts she had been given, and the sight to look past the basic to see something unique, once again I was given new life.

Yes, all the way from the initial meeting with my primary care doctor to the diagnosis to the surgery, the hand of God was continually present, blessing me with what I needed every step of the way. Now the cancer had been removed, and so we were on to the next step of the process—recovery from surgery and treatment to make sure that the cancer would not come back.

The Best Thing That Could Happen to Our Yard

I was only in the hospital for two days after the surgery. I was up and walking every few hours, the pain was minimal, and the charge nurse referred to me as the "rock star" of the floor. Jennifer brought the girls up to visit on Friday, and then they spent the night at a hotel in town before coming back Saturday to bring me home. The nurses loved having me there because I was so easy to care for, and the doctors were amazed at the progress I was making. We were still waiting for the results of the pathology, but so far everything was going as smoothly as it possibly could.

Saturday around noon I was loaded up into the van and taken home by my wonderful wife. As we pulled into the driveway, I was amazed to see all of the cars that were parked there. It turns out that the care team the church put together had decided to take the day to do a massive cleaning of the yard. They were weeding, picking up sticks and brush, mowing, and trimming. I was in awe, just seeing people out there cleaning my yard. It was a moving moment. Later on Jen would jokingly say that cancer was the best thing that could ever happen to our yard—it needed a lot TLC, and this great group of people gave it the care it needed.

I spent a lot of time the next few days napping. I was not able to sleep in the bed yet, so I slept in a recliner, which became my best friend. I also made myself get out and walk two to three times a day. It was great to feel the warm sun on my face and work up a little sweat even though I did not go all that far.

My first walk took me about six blocks, and on the way back I ran into a friend who was amazed I was moving as well as I was. She also expressed something that I had not thought of before. She mentioned how she was so paranoid of cancer that she had a hard time being around anyone who had it, not for fear of catching it, but rather because she had a very difficult time seeing what it did to people.

Later on I thought, *How many people are like that?* How many people avoid others because they fear what they might see? How many people avoid those who are sick because they are afraid something like that may happen to them?

This young lady said she could not come to church because seeing me would remind her of cancer, and since she was a smoker, lung cancer was a particular concern, and she did not want to be reminded of that.

Initially I was shocked by the conversation, but over time I came to realize that she was expressing a very human emotion—fear—and she was letting that fear dictate her life. I was at the opposite extreme at this point. I was so devoted to beating this cancer that fear was pushed so far back in my mind that it barely existed. I was much more focused on the blessings that I had been given that the fear I'd felt early on was starting to vanish.

I think that is so important in our lives. We are showered with blessings each and every day. Some of these blessings are huge, and some are so small that we only see them in hindsight. But when our eyes are opened, when we live knowing that we are loved, cared for, and needed by God and by others, then we can more clearly see the rich blessings we are given.

My blessings continued to grow. I was able to get out and walk more and more. I was able to spend time on the porch, watching my girls play in the yard and chase bubbles. I was able to enjoy sitting with my wife and sharing those special moments of just being together. And I was able to see the blessings I was given a little bit more clearly.

The first week home went quite quickly, and I was feeling great. On Friday I went into the office and led a wedding rehearsal. I returned on Saturday to do the wedding. It was wonderful to be able to do this ministry, but it wore me out. Luckily I had planned not to attend worship on Sunday, so I had another day to rest and recover.

The following week I started to ease back into a regular work schedule. I was there for half days most of the week. I also had a post-op appointment with my surgeon in Madison on that Wednesday. So Jennifer and I went up to meet with her. We met with her physician's assistant since she was still in surgery, which I understood very clearly after having taken extra surgery time from her a few weeks earlier. The PA said I was healing as well as possible. She also said that the scrapings of the lower lung were negative and that seven of the eleven lymph nodes had been infected, which meant there was a stopping point of the cancer at that time. The tumor on my heart had been totally encapsulated, so that was good news. She also said that because of the size of the tumor and its spreading to the lymph nodes, I was stage three A. This was, again, good news because the surgeon originally thought I would be stage three B. So I was given even more hope. The cancer was not as bad as expected. Stage three A is still not good, but it was not as far spread or as large as originally expected. So overall it was another good meeting, and now I was ready for the chemotherapy. I was scheduled to meet with the oncologist the next week to get set for that process.

My theology has always been extremely relational. I often teach and preach about the relational nature of God, how God comes to us and desires to build relationships with us, and how that relational nature then flows out of us. We are created to be in relationships with others, and it is in these relationships that we see the face of Christ more clearly.

But with all of the teaching and preaching I had done on this, experiencing it firsthand was quite different.

On the day I got home from the hospital, I experienced all my preaching and teaching in human form. The people that had gathered, the work they had done, the love they had shown to me and my family—I was overwhelmed.

Community had always been important to me, but this experience made it so much more concrete. Our church family reached out with arms of compassion that were much larger than I ever expected, and I was wrapped in an embrace of love that I will carry with me every day of my life.

The Return of the Mullet

The following week I met with the oncologist for the second time. He went over the surgeon's report with me and set up the schedule for chemo. The report had one piece of information that I had not been told before. It turns out that the first spot that was noticed on my lung, the one that started all of this, was not cancerous. Again, I saw a blessing here. The one thing that got the ball rolling and made my primary care doctor start running the tests was not cancer. But because she saw that spot, she ran the tests and found the other cancers that were in my body. The blessings abound.

My first chemo session was scheduled for three weeks later. The idea was that my body would heal up even more from the surgery and then I would be able to start chemo with as strong a system as possible. I would have four chemo sessions with twenty-one days between each session. Following the chemo I would then do some radiation. All the doctors agreed that I would have the whole kitchen sink thrown at me because of my age and the hope that we would get everything and not have to worry about it anymore.

Up to this point I really had no major concerns with everything we were doing. I was comfortable with the surgery, and I trusted the doctors. But now we were doing chemo, and this was the most nervous I had been. One of my aunts had had lung cancer but a different type. She was a smoker and had small-cell lung cancer. I had seen what she went through with chemo, and I was not looking forward to that. She had major nausea and was tired all the time. She lost all of her hair and a lot of weight. This was what I thought chemo would be like.

So I started to let people know via Facebook that I was going to start chemo, and the blessings of relationships came flying in. One of my old high school friends started to send me wigs in case I lost my hair. The first to arrive was the afro, followed soon by the mullet and the rock star. Such wonderful wigs being sent to a guy who really had very little hair to start with anyway. But it brought me laughter. I may have been entering a difficult time, but I was going to do it with a smile on my face.

When I met with the oncologist, I asked about losing my hair, and he said that with this type of chemo I probably would not lose any of it. The main reason I was asking was not because I feared losing it (I actually thought I would look good with a shaved head) but rather it was because I would have to find some way to let my girls know I would be bald. But, according to the doctor, that was not going to happen, so that conversation was avoided.

I then met with my chemo nurses, Robin and Tammy (who are some of the greatest saints in the world), and they set up a calendar as to when we would start, the prescriptions I would need filled, and how the day would progress.

I was going to be getting two different types of chemo, and because of the strength of these drugs, they were going to be giving me a lot of liquids because they did not want the drugs to sit in my kidneys for too long. Overall I was going to be in the clinic with an IV for six to eight hours for every session. My first thought was, *What am I going to do for that long a period of time?*

After all of the meetings, blood tests, and shots, I was finally done for the day. I was going to be returning in three weeks for the first session. At this point I was nervous but as ready as I could be.

God's Peace, God's Hope

Two weeks after surgery, I presided at two of our four worship services. It was wonderful to get back to what I love. The reception that I received was also amazing. When I came out and announced I was back, there was a huge round of applause at both of the services. Having that whole community, the body of Christ, surrounding me assured me that there are always others around to lift and support me, especially when I was having a hard time making it on my own. I was deeply moved.

The following week I was back in the pulpit. Writing a sermon and allowing myself to be open to what the Spirit has to say to me and to the congregation through me can sometimes be a daunting task. As I returned to the pulpit that weekend, I was feeling the pressure, but then the Spirit blew across me again. I was given a word, and that word became the focal point of my return sermon. The word was *peace.*

Peace—John 14:23–29

The past two months have been an experience to say the least. It has been a time filled with ups and downs. There have been the emotional extremes of tears to laughter in a matter of moments. It has been a time when I walked in some dark valleys and trekked to the highest peaks, a time when I have experienced and seen the face of Christ in amazing ways. It is through this journey that my eyes have been opened to the multitude of ways that I have seen God active in my live and in the lives of others. It has been an experience I will never forget.

One of the most amazing experiences happened on the day of surgery. Pastor Jennifer and I had arrived at the hospital a little before 5:30 in the morning. It had been a short night, but luckily we had driven up after confirmation the night before.

We didn't have to wait long before they lined all of us patients up and took us back into these little cubicles. They had me put on one of those wonderful little gowns with the natural air-conditioning slit up the back. Then they came and took vitals, drew blood, all of that fun stuff.

After we got settled in, Pastor Pedro from the synod office popped his head in. He sat and talked, shared scripture, and prayed.

It was getting closer now.

At this point, I still felt rather relaxed, considering everything that was about to happen. Pedro left, and another friend who had driven out from Minnesota popped his head in. He was only there a couple of minutes, and then came the surgical team. Doctors, nurses, anesthesiologists, just piles of people coming in and getting me ready to go. Then it was time, so I gave Pastor Jennifer a kiss, and off I went.

As I was being wheeled down that very white hallway, the nerves started to set in. I started thinking all of those "what ifs." You know those questions that pop in your head and bring the deepest, darkest fears to the surface.

Then, as they opened the doors to the operating room and were about to wheel me in, it came to me.

Peace.

Peace, Erik, I am here.

Peace, I am with you.

Peace, I am leading you into this place.

That peace, that sensation that overtook me at that moment, was exactly what I needed, for I knew I was in good hands, and I don't mean only those of that very talented surgeon and her team. But rather I was in the good hands of the God who led me into that operating room and gave me the peace I needed at that time.

Peace.

Have you ever had a moment like that, a time when you were feeling a little anxious, nervous, or upset? Then, in the midst of that anxiety, this calming peace overcame you, and you felt that presence, that sense of comfort, fill your entire being?

On that early morning that gift of peace sustained me at a time when I needed it the most. It was the gift of knowing that I was not alone but rather God was right there, leading the way into the operating room, carrying me.

Today, in the gospel, we hear Jesus give us the assurance of that peace in our lives. This is taking place near the end of his ministry. It is the last night he has with his disciples, and so he has gathered them around, and he teaches them one last time.

During this teaching he tries to let them know that he will be leaving them soon, but even though he is going, he is not leaving them alone. No, Jesus, their friend, their rabbi, their LORD, he is not going to abandon them. He is sending an advocate, the Holy Spirit, to be with them until his return. But he doesn't stop there.

Jesus goes on and says, "Peace I leave with you, My Peace I give to you."

Now the peace Jesus is talking about here is a little different than we might think of today. It is not a peace like end of a war or battle. It is not a peace like the laying down of arms. But rather peace for Jesus is two things. It is comfort for the troubled heart and courage in the midst of fear.

Comfort and courage.

These are two things we desperately need in our lives. Comfort and courage: this is what gets us through the dark valleys of life that we sometimes stumble into.

Comfort and courage: it is the blessing of being able to face head on whatever struggles we have and knowing we are not doing so alone.

Comfort and courage: it is the gift of peace, of God's peace, and the assurance of God's presence in our lives.

You see, that is why Jesus is talking to his disciples about peace on this night. He is about to make that walk, that Holy-Week walk, all the way to Golgotha. But before he goes, he wants his disciples, he wants us, to make sure we know that he will not ever leave us alone. Christ will always be with us.

No matter where we go, no matter what we do, Christ will be there. He will shower us with his comfort, his courage, and his peace, all so we know that we are his children, and we always will be.

To put an exclamation point on his teaching, Jesus then lives out his gift of peace during his last days. For throughout the events of his arrest, trial, and crucifixion, as well as in the resurrection, Jesus embodies the peace he offers here. He lives out this peace as he gives his all so that we might live and live eternally. Yes, Jesus wants the disciples to know that even though he is leaving them in human form, he is not orphaning them. He wants us to know that the love he has for all his children, for all of us, is so great that he will come and give us the peace, the comfort, the courage we need to make it through whatever the world throws at us.

I have no doubt that this was the peace I was given as I was wheeled into that operating room—the comfort and courage of God as I went into surgery.

I remember being wheeled into that operating room, now more relaxed than I was when I was wheeled down that white hallway. I was told to help move my body from the bed to this cold operating table. I remember lying back on this stainless steel, and I felt the nurse strap my feet to the table.

But that's it. That's all I remember.

With the exception of the sensation of comfort, of peace, surrounding me.

Yes, it was that peace that gave me the assurance that all would be all right, and it was. Yes, God promises he will walk through life with us, every step of the way. He will grant us the peace that we need to celebrate this gift of life and share it with others so we can go out into the world, trusting in the fact that our God is a God filled with love and compassion. A God who blesses us with peace, comfort, and courage, and he does all of this out of the great love that he has for each and every one of us, his children, his beloved. Yes, he does all this for you.

Providing Humor for Others

Not long after my first trip back into the pulpit, I had another meeting with my oncologist. We were preparing for me to start my chemo sessions, but I also got some interesting news about my cancer.

The oncologist had received an e-mail from the medical team at the University of Wisconsin. They had run some tests and confirmed that the cancer was caused by a genetic mutation. It turns out that the tumor was caused by EML4-Alk chromosomal translocation. This occurs in less than 3 percent of the people who have non-small-cell lung cancer and usually occurs in non-smokers. There is a company developing a drug that targets this gene rearrangement, and the clinic trials have had nearly a 90 per cent success rate.

It is very rare to have this, and the doctor actually laughed when I said, "Yeah, I keep telling people I am unique."

This did not change anything for my treatment at that time because there was nothing approved by the FDA or in trials in the area to treat this. But he did say that if there were a relapse, then there probably would be a new treatment that would be beneficial. The way he explained it, chemo is like taking a sledgehammer to kill a bug on the table; you will kill the bug and destroy the table as well. The new therapy would target the bug only and not harm the table.

The doctor agreed with me when I said the prayer is that the chemo and radiation will work, but if there is a relapse, there is a very good plan B in the works. The blessings of having a plan B cannot be overlooked.

The night before my first chemo session I was busy downloading tunes for my iPod. I thought that if I was going to be sitting around for six to eight hours, I should have some new tunes to go with me. As I was scrolling through some new artists I had not heard of before, I found one song titled, "Healing Begins." Immediately I played a sample, and I was hooked. The major theme had to do with how it is only through brokenness that healing can take place. This became the theme song for my first week of chemo and overall for my time of treatment.

Later that night my wife and girls gave me what Sierra called my "Chemo Care Kit." Jennifer had taken the girls shopping to keep them involved in the process in a healthy way, and they purchased snacks, Sudoku puzzles, and other trinkets to keep me busy for the day. It was moving, sitting there, knowing I was about to get treated for a deadly disease and seeing my wife, five-year-old, and one-year-old hand me a care package. It was as if they were saying, "This will be a walk in the park. Here is something to have fun with while you are away." There are still times today that I look over one of the items that was in the Chemo Care Kit, and I get teary, for the faith and support that my family has shown is utterly amazing. Having this support, having this love, is a blessing that cannot be overstated.

So I was up and with the nurse by 9:30 on Monday morning. I had my iPod, Kindle, DVDs of *The West Wing*, and Chemo Care Kit from my family. I also had Jennifer stop for a mocha on the way in. *Might was well make the best of it,* I thought.

It began with an IV of fluids followed by six or so different IV bags. They only had to stick me once, so that was positive, and the whole process really was not all that tough—just sitting there, taking in the chemo, and trying to make the time pass.

Around noon Jennifer brought lunch up, so I was able to talk with her as we shared our subs. She then left to get the girls from school, and I was about to start a DVD when two members of the congregation came in.

One of them was our doctor friend who had come to Madison with me, and the other was a seven-year cancer survivor. Both of them brought a sense of humor that was much needed. As soon as they arrived, Sue, the cancer survivor, pulled out some knitting and said, "Here, hold this."

Earlier in the day my mother-in-law had posted on Facebook that I should have taken up knitting because it would have helped to pass the time. So Sue decided this would be a good time to fake a picture and send it to her with me pretending to learn how to knit.

Ah, the blessings of humor. Without it life would be so dull.

Nancy and Sue stayed for a few hours. We talked, laughed, and I was reminded again about the importance of community and relationships.

Halfway through the treatment, right before they were going to give me the second of the chemo drugs I was taking, the nurse came in and said, "Now, I'm going to give you an IV version of a water pill. The reason we do this is that this medicine is very potent and we don't want it staying in your kidneys very long." So she gave me the shot, then, as she was about to leave, said, "Oh, and with that shot you will have to go to the bathroom about every fifteen minutes, that's why we unplugged your IV."

And so, the second round of humor with Nancy and Sue started. They would sit and talk with me as they watched the clock, just waiting for me to get up and go. After the sixth trip to the restroom, Nancy and Sue even got the nurses laughing at me, or with me, depending on who you ask.

After they left I completed my first chemo session. I was one quarter of the way done with this part of the treatment, and I could actually see the end line. This may not be fun, it may not be all that easy, but the end result would be what we were looking for—a cancer-free future.

No Mullet Needed (My Wife Rejoices)

The first week after the chemo treatment was much smoother than I ever expected. The side effects were quite minimal, the doctor was right, and I maintained all the hair I had, which meant the mullet and afro stayed in their packaging, and after six days I was almost at 100 percent.

The three minor side effects I had were a small bit of nausea (which was well controlled with some great meds), being tired, especially days three to five after the treatment (naps are a blessing!), and the one that surprised me—the chemo hiccups. It turns out that the drugs I was given and the steroid that went with it can cause hiccups in some people. I got that one. On Tuesday night I got the hiccups four times, each round lasting about an hour. Luckily I was able to get a new med that I could take if it happened again.

On Tuesday I went in for my weekly blood draw, and all of the panels looked great. My system had been adapting to the chemo extremely well, and I was up and starting exercise once again. During this time I was continually amazed at how blessed I had been through this entire ordeal. I felt good, and I was full of hope that these treatments would wipe out any cancer cells that were hiding in my system!

After going through all of this, I had come up with a couple of ministry ideas. The first one I put into action was the Cancer Prayer Support Group. As I had seen how important the blessing of community was to me, I wanted to make sure that others could have that blessing in their lives as well. So this was a group that started meeting twice a month to be there for one another. We are a support group but also a group that is grounded in prayer—praying for ourselves, our families, medical teams, and for others who are battling this disease as well.

For me, another one of the blessings that came out of all of this was being able to meet others where they are with a renewed vision. Being able to be with people, to sit with them during their struggles and trials, has been a gift of mine. But now I came at it from a different angle. I was in their shoes, and they were in mine. This gave my ministry a renewed energy.

Three weeks later I started round two of chemo. The morning started with another blood draw, which had become one of the weekly joys I got to endure during this time, then a meeting with the oncologist, followed by seven hours of having fluids and chemo pumped into my system.

In many ways the second session was like the first. Jennifer brought me lunch, Sue and Nancy came and harassed me, and another member of the congregation, Steve, came to visit as well. Steve was on the call committee when we came to this congregation, and since day one the two of us have hit it off. His wife refers to us as brothers because we have such similar tastes, styles, and senses of humor. His visit helped to brighten the morning in a wonderful way. And, once again, the chemo did its job. But this time I was in a room with other chemo patients, and the church was present.

It turns out that during this time there were four of us from our congregation going through chemo. I was by far the youngest, and I was the one who had the longest treatment regimen for the day. On this particular day, the other three were all with me at one point or another, two of them getting treatment, the third setting up a treatment schedule.

During this time I was reminded again about the value of community. Those of us who were going through treatment all knew that we were facing a difficult battle with cancer, but as we sat there, with IVs pumping chemo through our bodies, we also knew that these were battles we faced with others. We had never been alone, and even in the dark times when it felt like we were alone, God would reach out his hand and touch us in an amazing way. The blessing of community, the blessing of being part of this great body called the church, shines through even the darkest of valleys that we may face.

❧

After round two of chemo, I was reminded again of what a blessing we have in modern medicine. Throughout this entire time, I never went through the nasty nausea that so many people experience. Because of all the advances in medicine, the chemo can often do what it needs to without tearing the rest of the body apart. It was also at this time that I learned more about the new med in final trials that related to my specific genetic mutation cancer. It turns out that our plan B had so much success in trials that it skipped from stage-one trials to final trials. The success rate was running at about 90 percent, and many people were very excited about this new drug.

For me, what I saw was another blessing. Just in case plan A of chemo and radiation didn't work, a door was being opened for another healing avenue. God's endowing people with the knowledge and foresight to develop medicines that specifically attack these cancerous cells is an amazing blessing indeed.

This also opened my eyes to the future. Up to this point, I was afraid to look to the future. I always had that dark little place in my mind that said, "If you look to the future, you will get burned. Don't be surprised if you don't make it too far." But now I had even more hope, and so I started dreaming about the future again. We made plans for some trips, and I saw the blessings of living with hope with a renewed vigor.

I prepared to do radiation so that the healing process could continue in new ways. It was during this time that I came to another realization, probably one of the biggest I had up to this point.

Three years earlier my father had been diagnosed with bladder cancer. He had gone to Mayo Clinic to have surgery and be treated, and during this time he mentioned to them that he had some problems with his hands. They ran a few tests on him, and he was eventually diagnosed with ALS, Lou Gehrig's Disease.

Amyotrophic lateral sclerosis is a disease that eats away at the body, and there is a very low survival rate. The majority of people diagnosed with ALS die within eighteen months of diagnosis.

Dad took this diagnosis extremely hard. He had been a very outgoing man who loved to talk and share stories over coffee. Even though he lived in Montana and I was in Wisconsin, we would talk three to four times a week. But as soon as he was diagnosed, it was like everything was switched off. We stopped talking as much, and the joy and excitement that was always on his face seemed to disappear. The last few months of his life seemed to be more of an endurance rather than a living.

When I was diagnosed with cancer, I knew it was serious, even life-threatening. But instead of taking the road my dad took, shutting down and shutting people out, I decided to go the opposite route. I started to reconnect with more old friends. I wrote about my experiences on a blog and tried to celebrate every day as the gift it was.

In doing all of this, my joy for living was taken to another level. I was able to see the blessings of God more clearly each day, and even on the days when I was struggling, when I was having a hard time physically or emotionally, I was always able to see outside of the pit that I was in because of the love with which I was showered.

That is how it works sometimes. Sometimes we need to enter into the valleys of life in order to enjoy the mountaintops all the more. Sometimes we need to enter into struggles in order to enjoy the regular and the mundane. Sometimes we need to cry in order to experience joy.

There cannot be a resurrection until there is a death. But when the resurrection comes, when the light breaks through the darkness, it is impossible to miss the multitude of blessings that surround us. Blessings of life, relationships, love, compassion—the list goes on and on.

Twenty-Five Years

The rest of the chemo sessions went as smoothly as the first two. I was continually amazed at how easy chemo actually was for me. The nausea remained minimal, the chemo hiccups disappeared, and the biggest problem I had was getting enough sleep the first few days after the chemo. The steroids I took kept me awake at night, but naps kept me going, and I was able to work and celebrate the gifts of life as I went through this treatment.

I met with the oncologist before my last session and went through the follow-up plan. The next step was to have radiation. Then in three months I would have my first post-treatment CT scan. These scans would occur every three months for the first three years, every six months for years four and five, and then annually after that.

So as we were about to part ways, I finally asked the question I had been afraid to ask.

What is the relapse rate for this type of cancer?

He responded by saying there is at least a 50 percent chance that the cancer could return.

I know that seems like a good chance it could return, but, again, I heard something different. I heard that there was almost a 50 percent chance that it would not return. I also had done some research, and it was only a few years ago when they had not done any treatments following lung cancer surgery, but once they started using the treatments that I received, the five-year survival rate jumped by about 60 to 70 percent.

So I finished the chemo treatments and then was headed off to another part of the hospital—the cancer care center where they gave radiation therapy.

My first meeting was with the doctor to discuss what radiation is and how they would administer it. He went through the process: I would be scanned, marked, and come in daily for treatments that would only take ten to fifteen minutes per session. He talked about what parts of my body would be focused on, and then he mentioned something that stuck with me.

He said that if they had to target over my heart, where the thymoma (the tumor that was discovered on my heart) was, then there would be a chance in twenty-five years I would need to have heart surgery.

All I heard was twenty-five years.

Again, it was a sign of hope—hope that I was going to beat this and I was going to be around for a long time after the treatments ended.

I was introduced to the rest of the radiation staff and brought in to get a CT scan. The purpose of this scan was to line up exactly where they wanted to target the radiation. Then they plucked some hair off of my chest and made a mark with a blue Sharpie in the middle of my chest and then one on both sides. This was to make sure that I was in the same position every time I came in for treatment. They were also marks that would be on me for the next seven weeks with small pieces of tape over them to protect them when I showered. The team I met was wonderful, and I knew I was in good hands for my radiation sessions.

So I began the last leg of my treatment journey.

After I went through all of the prep work for the radiation treatments, and before they started, I took a little trip. As I had been going through my chemo treatments, I knew that I wanted to meet up with some old friends, so I planned a drive to the Twin Cities. I called it my I-survived-chemo gathering and invited everyone in the area, as well as some nowhere near the cities, to meet up and have a night to just catch up.

So on a Thursday afternoon, I left home and drove to the cities. I met up with Mitch, who had come up from a small town in southern Minnesota to be there. We had dinner and went to a local watering hole for the night.

Then people started showing up. Throughout the night a number of friends—spanning high school, college, seminary, and former church members—came together. It was one of the most diverse gatherings I had been a part of in a long time, and it was a wonderfully uplifting evening.

The next day I went to a college roommate's cabin to celebrate the birthday of another roommate. I was seeing people I had not seen in years, and I had a wonderful time refreshing those relationships.

This time away and the time with old friends reinvigorated me for the final step of the treatment that was awaiting me. I was ready to tackle this last stage head on and make sure that there were no more little cancer cells hiding in me.

Getting Zapped

I returned from my trip on Sunday afternoon, and on Wednesday I was ready to go. I went in to the radiation center for a 2:00 p.m. appointment, and they brought me into the room where I would get all my treatments. I was told that every week they would take X-rays of me to make sure they were shooting in the correct areas. Then they had me take off my shirt, lie down on the table, and start the process. They adjusted the sheet underneath me so all of my marks lined up and then started the session.

The machine had a big arm on it, and at the top of the arm was a large circular head that shot out the radiation. The arm and head rotated around the table I was lying on, and they shot the radiation into me from five different angles. Overall the process only took about ten minutes. On this first day they took a little longer, making sure everything was lined up right and that the marks were still in the right place. After about forty minutes, I was done with day one.

I also learned that day that I would be having twenty-five sessions. These sessions would take place Monday through Friday, and the only days off would be weekends and holidays. Twenty-five sessions—five weeks—and then I was done with treatment. I knew I could handle this last leg of the treatment journey.

The next day I showed up at 8:30 a.m., and we were off and running. This was my regularly scheduled time for these sessions, and I enjoyed being able to get everything done before heading into work. The nursing staff was great, and on the days I had to bring Sierra in with me, they would play with her and load her up on tons of sugar—a great way to start the day.

One of the blessings that I received at this time was the ten minutes of solitude I got while receiving the treatments. During this time, when no one could enter the room I was in, I was able to slow down and spend time in prayer. This time of conversation with God was amazing, as it got me to focus on all of the things that I was grateful for in life. I spent the majority of my time thanking God for my family, friends, and all the doctors and nurses who were working with me to beat this disease. I spent a lot of time praying for others who were battling different illnesses as well. Being able to have this time in prayers of thanksgiving while receiving treatment was a blessing to me, for it reminded me to see all of the blessings I have been given and to look at the positive side of life.

Returning to the Starting Point

The treatments went on without any troubles, and I was excited to be done. During the last week of the sessions, I had another regularly scheduled six-month appointment with my primary care doctor. I have to admit I was really looking forward to this appointment.

The reason I was so excited for this appointment was that I wanted to thank her for all that she had done. Over the past six months, trying though they may have been, I was amazingly grateful for this doctor and all she had done for me. What's more, all the doctors I had met over the past six months were impressed by her as well. Some even said that it was a rarity for a doctor to do the follow-up tests that she had done, for many would have waited, and in doing so the cancer would have been much worse than it was.

On Monday morning I went to my regular radiation treatment, and when I was done, I headed over to see my doctor. I had brought a gift for her, a nice bottle of wine since I had heard that she was a bit of a connoisseur. I knew that giving her a gift to thank her was the right thing to do. Again, this goes back to my relational theology—it is about God and the people we encounter on this journey of life. So taking that extra little step, saying the thank you, giving the gift, all of it helps to empower and build up the other, and I think that is part of our calling—to love and serve others and care for them just as God has cared for us.

I went in and did all of the regular testing—weight (still have to work on that one), blood pressure, pulse, etc. All looked pretty good, so the nurse left. A few minutes later, in came the doctor. She started by asking about the second tumor that was found on my heart, the thymoma. The big question was how long that had been there, for it was probably years. Then I was able to profess my gratitude to her, give her the gift, and say, "Without you, there is a good chance this would not have been caught in time. You helped to save my life, and I will always be grateful."

The rest of the appointment was fairly uneventful. We went through the last six months, made some plans for the future (exercise and weight loss at the top of this list), and set up the next appointment.

A quick note on the weight loss bit. This is something I have struggled with for years, but now my struggle has an addition to it—a mental block to weight loss. You see, in my little warped mind, I think that if I am losing weight, then the cancer is back, since weight loss in one of the signs of a tumor. So not only do I have to change my diet and get exercise, but I also need to convince myself that weight loss does not mean the cancer is back. I am continuing to work on that.

Luckily I had already started the working out portion of the program, joining a class at the YMCA that starts at 5:15 in the morning. The AM Fit Club, it is called, and it has made me plenty sore. But, hey, it is a good pain, according to my instructor. So now I just need to get over the mental block and put down that yummy doughnut.

The final radiation session arrived. On that Wednesday morning, I stopped at McDonald's and picked up mochas for the radiation staff. They had been so wonderful to me, and to be the first one they saw in the morning, I thought they might need a little extra kick.

I remember walking in, and the first thing the nurse asked was if I was doing my happy dance. Everyone there was excited for me because all of them knew what a big deal it was: six months of surgery, chemo, and radiation—that is a lot for a body, and a mind, and a soul, to handle.

So we did our last session, and I was even offered a kiss from one of the techs for the gift of the coffee (see, it is all about relationships), and then I was given a certificate for the completion of the radiation treatments. It was just a little thing, but little things can make a big impact.

I had another meeting with the doctor where we set up a schedule for follow-up visits, and he encouraged me to keep up with the exercise plan and not be afraid of weight loss meaning the cancer was back. Then I was done.

Done.

The next morning I did not need to see a doctor or nurse.

The next week I did not need to give blood.

In fact, I had an entire month off until my first quarterly CT scan.

What was I going to do with all this free time?

Six months is not a long period of time in our lives. But during this time a lot can happen, and those six months, well, they were amazing for me. I experienced just about every emotion I could. I met tons of doctors and nurses, I gave a lot of blood, and was stuck with needles galore (I continue to thank God for having good veins that were easy to stick). I had seen a lot in six months, and now that part of the journey was over.

I was done.

Celebrating the Blessings

Throughout this entire time, the treatments went as smoothly as they possibly could. Through my blog I was able to inform and educate the congregation on what cancer treatments are like, and I was reminded of what a blessing the body of Christ, the church, truly is.

But the biggest part of this journey, for me, was the way that God continued to open my eyes to the blessings around me. Every step of this journey, even the diagnosis, was filled with blessings. There were some times when it was difficult to see the blessings, but they were there. These blessings helped me to see the face of Christ in others, sometimes in the most unexpected places, and through these blessings I was continually lifted up in arms of grace and love.

I am now looking forward to the future. I have had three post-treatment CT scans, and they have all been clean; there was no cancer to be seen. I will continue to have CT scans to make sure that the cancer has not returned, and we are all hopeful that since the treatments went as well as they did that the scans will be negative. As of now I am a one-year cancer survivor and was recently told that the protocols for follow-up treatments have changed. No longer will I be having scans every three months for three years, and then every six months for two more years with five years being the magic number for a very small chance of recurrence. With the new protocols I will have one more year of scans every four months, and once I hit the two-year mark, the chance of recurrence is minimal. Another blessing—the treatments do work. I have no doubt that there will still be times of fear, times of doubt, times of questioning, but I also know that these times will be swallowed up with the blessings that God will continue to shower upon me through his body.

I know this because that is what God does—he empowers, blesses, and cares for his children, and he does all of this out of the love he has for us. That is the greatest blessing of all.

1-1-14

Comfort & courage what we need in our lives face things head on not doing so alone